Anti Inflammatory Diet

The Ultimate Diet Guide That Will Help You Lose Weight, Reverse Aging, Eliminate Pain, and Restore Your Overall Health

By

Hannah Parkes

© 2016

Copyright & Disclaimer:

Table of Contents

Introduction

If you are reading this, chances are, you are done. You are done feeling groggy and run-down. You are done being overweight and overwhelmed. Read this book if you are ready to begin working on a diet that is going to make the biggest change you can imagine in your life.

The anti inflammatory diet is not a diet that focuses on just one area. It is not a starve-yourself plan. Honestly, it can hardly even be called a diet. The anti inflammatory diet is more of a lifestyle change. A change that, if done right, can leave you feeling happier, healthier, and ready to take on the world.

The anti inflammatory diet focuses on reducing unwanted inflammation in the body. Sure, inflammation can be fantastic and helpful when it comes to healing bumps and bruises, but it can also wreak havoc. Inflammation can cause pre-mature aging and accelerate the aging process by preventing stem cells from performing in a way that they need to. It can also be the cause of increased weight gain and instability. Inflammation can leave you feeling groggy and tired, making clear decisions and mindfulness impossible. On top of all that, allowing inflammation, weight gain, and unhealthy digestion to continue unchecked increases chances of cancer, arthritis, and other degenerative diseases.

When you look at everything together, the choice appears to be simple. Make a change for the better. This book contains details on inflammation, the anti inflammatory diet, and other lifestyle chances you can make to improve upon your own well being. It gives you details on the best and worst foods you can eat when you focus on inflammation. This comprehensive quick-start guide should be everything you need to start working on your lifestyle change today.

Chapter 1

What is Inflammation?

Inflammation is a response from your immune system to help heal your body. This can be useful when you have an injury or actual issue within your body. It increases white blood cell counts and gives the body the ability to protect organs and tissue from outside invaders. Inflammation is exactly what it sounds like. It is the swelling and redness of tissues, muscles, and other parts of your body.

The issue with inflammation is that it can be too active. It can work when and where it isn't supposed to. It can over-load our bodies, joints, organs, and lives with too much swelling. One of the most common examples of inflammation causing unnecessary swelling is arthritis. Your body isn't listening to you. You need to make it stop, and take control of your own inflammation.

Your body goes through a lot on a daily basis. It takes on and battles toxins, conquers stress, does everything you ask it to, digests everything you put in your mouth, and much more. The human body was not meant to conquer as many un-natural products as it does today. From smog to stress to processed foods, it's no wonder inflammation is a huge problem. Take on this anti inflammatory diet as a tool to help you change your life for the better.

Chapter 2
Benefits of an Anti Inflammatory Diet

Lower Inflammation Levels

As the title of the anti inflammatory diet suggests, the main goal is to lower your inflammation. It is intended to keep your body from having an inflammatory reaction when it isn't necessary. As you lower the toxins that your digestion system has to deal with you give your body the permission it needs to be healthy and take care of itself the way it needs to. You will begin to eliminate that knee-jerk reaction that is inflammation.

Use the anti-inflammatory diet to take some of the strain off of your immune system. You may feel fine (or not) and still have high levels of inflammation in your body. This inflammation can wreak havoc.

Weight Loss

This diet, or rather, lifestyle change, isn't promising that you will lose weight quickly, or even at all. Instead, is focuses on the overall healthiness of *you*. This may, and for most people does, mean weight loss. It gives you the tools you need to make conscious decisions about your body and increases the healthiness of your digestion.

If your digestive tract is healthy, you are at a better place for losing weight. It helps your body know to eliminate the sugars and other things it normally stores up in fat cells. The human body was built in nature, not with processed foods and daily toxins. The weight loss you will experience when moving your life towards an anti inflammatory diet will be the type of weight loss that sticks. If you stick to this program, you will consistently feel good and in-turn, look good. The anti inflammatory diet isn't about starving yourself, it's about eating and doing the right things to help your overall health.

Increased Energy

How long have you felt down in the dumps? Do you find it super hard to get yourself out of bed in the mornings and off of the couch in the evenings? How is anyone supposed to take care of themselves when they feel ragged and run-down?

The anti inflammatory diet is created to help you improve your energy levels. If your body is fighting off toxins and working to focus on unnecessary inflammation, how is it supposed to give you energy? As you give your body the right foods and ingredients to take care of itself, it will begin to take care of you. Your digestive tract will be able to absorb the vitamins and minerals you need to keep you going. Your brain will be able to focus and push the right energy to the right places. If your energy is increased, how much more could you get done?

Lower Pain Levels

Aches, pains, and headaches . . . oh my! The anti inflammatory diet can help with all of this! The inflammation in our bodies and toxins makes it hard for our immune system to do any extra work. Follow the anti inflammation diet and you should see these pains go away. You will be giving your body what it needs and answering the calls that it makes when it comes up with indescribable pain in the gut. Give yourself the right nutrition and I promise you will see tremendous difference in your pain levels.

Are your joints bothering you? The anti inflammatory diet helps your body slow does the inflammation and irritation you are feeling. Feeling weird pains in your gut? This could be from inflammation and over-working in the digestion tract. You can make sure that doesn't happen and make your tummy a whole lot happier. Headaches galore? Dehydration, lack of proper nutrition, and inflammation can be three major causes of headaches. The anti-inflammatory diet and suggestions made in this book are going to be geared towards fixing that.

Reversed Aging

When your body isn't working properly, your stem cells aren't going to work either. Are bodies are kept young and fresh with the help of stem cells replacing old, worn-out, ones. However, these stem cells need help to work properly and stay together. When stem cells stop being produced, your body begins to age, rapidly. Keep yourself young with the anti inflammatory diet. This means that your wrinkles and rusty-bones may just be a thing of the past. Healthier people are happier people, and happier people look younger.

Skin, Hair, and Nails

Have you ever noticed your hair falling out? Is your skin constantly dry? Do you nails crack or look disgusting? All of these and other issues with the skin, hair, and nails, are often signs of poor nutrition. That means that either something is missing in your diet, or something is not getting absorbed into your body in the way it needs to be.

The anti inflammatory diet includes conversations about supplements and the best diet combination for your diet. It tells you what to eat and what to avoid. When you eat the right things, you are giving you hair, skin, and nails, room to grow and improve. You are feeding them the right ingredients. When you avoid the bad foods and practices, you stop poisoning yourself. You are able to make it so that the right nutrients are absorbed and sent to the right part of your body.

Overall Optimized Health

It's clear that the anti inflammatory diet can provide a good picture of overall optimized health. It will make you feel better if you use it to help change your lifestyle. It can help safe-guard against cancers and other diseases. It is not fool proof, it is not magical. It is simply the practice of treating your body the way it deserves to be treated. In the coming chapters, I will discuss ways in which you can optimize yourself and reach an optimal health. Do the right thing for your body and it will be nicer to you.

Chapter 3

Put Your Dukes up! Fight against Inflammation

You may be thinking to yourself, that is all awesome, but what do I do to fight against this inflammation? There are a few very important elements to this battle. Here are the basic guidelines you need to follow as you work to reduce the inflammation in your body and make your life better. Remember, the anti-inflammatory diet is more than just a diet. It is a change in your lifestyle to improve everything about your body. These basics are about making you feel better everywhere, giving you more energy and reducing inflammation.

Calorie Count

The anti inflammatory diet is not a diet that aims to starve you. It is not about reducing caloric intake drastically. Instead, it wants you to get the right foods in your body. If you pay attention to what you are doing with your food, you can maintain a relatively normal caloric intake. Most people find that they can maintain a diet between 2,000 and 3,000 calories. This is not a one-size-fits-all standard. If you find that you are meeting your calorie goal, but still not losing weight or feeling any better, then reduce your caloric intake. If you are more active and have a healthier metabolism, then you have a higher caloric intake. The most important aspect of managing your calories is paying attention to yourself. Decide how you feel and keep your calorie intake where you need it to be. Although your caloric intake is important in the anti-inflammatory diet, it is by no means the most important aspect.

Carbs

Carbohydrates take a lot to process and often end up getting stored in fat cells where we don't want them on our bodies. You should eat between 200g and 300g of carbs a day. Women should make sure they are at the lower end of that spectrum while men can eat a little bit more.

Water

Make sure that you are always drink plenty of water. Water can make or break your diet. If you don't drink enough water each day you may experience any of all of the following symptoms, the more dehydrated you are the worse it can be: Fatigue, dizziness, mood swings, muscle cramps, chills, foggy thinking, poor concentration, constipation, headaches, joint pain, and much more. Drinking water can help keep your inflammation levels down, your pain levels down, and toxins flushed out of your body. If you do everything else that this diet asks you to do, but you do not drink enough water, you may prevent yourself from reaping any of the rewards. *Remember*, your urine color is a good indicator of how much water you should be drinking. You should always strive for a light colored urine. If it is as dark as apple juice or tea, you need to drink more. Strong smelling urine is also a good sign of dehydration. To be an active participant in the anti-inflammatory diet, make sure you are drinking plenty of water. Water is also an active part of your skin, drinking more of it can help with your goal to look younger. If the skin has the right hydration it can prevent cracking and wrinkles and even reverse some wrinkles through rejuvenation.

Vitamins and Minerals

A well rounded diet can work wonders for your diet. Make sure you are getting all of the right vitamins and minerals. Getting this combination right can mean positive results for your inflammation levels.

- Vitamin A – This antioxidant can help protect your body against free radicals and other diseases. It has strong anti-inflammatory effects. It can help with the digestion in your intestine, your lungs, and your skin. This is a hard one to find in food, so if you really want the helpful effects of vitamin A, take a supplement to help you along.

- Vitamin B6 – This vitamin also fights that nasty inflammation. It can be found it foods like beef, turkey, vegetables, and fish. Make sure you eat something that has Vitamin B6 in it daily to replenish your stores. Vitamin B6 will especially help you if you suffer from any arthritis or joint pain.

- Vitamin C – Vitamin C is commonly known for strengthening the immune system to keep you from getting sick. This is an important aspect in your health. Oranges, citrus fruits, broccoli, and some other vegetables have good stores of Vitamin C. This is a positive anti-oxidant that helps fight for you that comes with some anti-inflammatory effects. Make sure you get plenty of this in what you eat, if not, take a supplement.

- Vitamin D – This supplement has proven results in decreasing inflammation. It might even help lower your cancer risks.

- Vitamin E – Vitamin E is commonly found in nuts, seeds, and leafy greens. Make sure you get plenty of this to help you with your anti-inflammatory goals.

- Vitamin K – Like Vitamin E, Vitamin K is found in leafy greens. It is even known to help reduce the risk of blot clots, which will keep you happy, healthy, and on your feet.

- Coenzyme q10 – This in an antioxidant and can be found in things like salmon, beef liver, olive oil, peanuts, and avocado. It is believed to have anti-inflammatory benefits and be linked to some tasty meals.

- Glutathione – Much like Vitamin A, this is a free-radical fighter. This means that Glutathione protects your body with some anti-inflammatory benefits thrown in. This can be found in avocados, spinach, tomatoes, garlic, apples, and asparagus.

- Omega 3 Fatty Acids – These are found in oily fish and supplements. They help reduce inflammation in the body and make you feel much better.

Some studies suggest that a baseline A-Z vitamin supplement may help you all around with your anti-inflammatory diet goals. This is a positive route to take. Make sure you check and balance what you are eating and what you are taking with how you feel each day. Deficiencies in any of these vitamins cause inflammation and pain in the body. If you want to feel better, this is area you want to pay close attention to.

Write It All Down

A really good way to make sure that you are following this diet correctly, is to keep a journal. However, don't just keep a food journal with calorie counts, keep a feelings journal. Each day, write down everything you are eating and drinking and how you are feeling. I promise you, this will be a crucial step in you feeling better. You will begin to notice that as you feel better, the foods, waters, and minerals are balanced. You will also notice that when you feel worse it is usually because you ate something off of the no-go list. Like I said at the beginning of the book, this diet is more than just a diet, it is a way of life. Over time, you will notice that your skin and aging areas will look better, your muscles and pains will feel better, and you will be happier. Write about it so that you remember why you started in the first place.

Chapter 4
Foods to Avoid

In case you hadn't noticed, food is an important part of this diet. The anti inflammatory diet is about more than just counting calories and getting the right nutrients. Make sure you avoid the following foods, especially in excess. Some of them may seem harmless, but they are not taking care of your body like you need. They will cause more inflammation, pain, and digestion issues than they will solve.

Sugar – I know it can be hard to curve those sweet cravings, but it's important to avoid it, especially those processed sugars. Sugars and sweeteners can show up under all kinds of different names. Often, they are fall under names that end in "ose," like sucrose or dextrose.

Dairy – Milk is designed by nature to make baby cows gain weight. It makes it so they can grow up rapidly before they start feeding on their regular diet of grasses and natural foods. Dairy is extremely inflammatory and can wreck your diet and how you are feeling. In addition to this, the dairy that we consume every day is more processed which just continues to add inflammatory attributes and makes you feel even more miserable.

Gluten and Refined Breads – Gluten is a man-made substance that resides in almost every refined grain. It makes you feel worse and causes inflammation and irritation. This much processing is not what your body was made to digest. Gluten can be found in bread, pizza, pasta, and even cereal. This is one you want to be especially careful on.

Processed and Commercially-Fed Meats – When these animals are raised, they are kept in captivity, fed food that they aren't meant to eat, and kept alive with hormones and anti-biotics. When meats like pepperoni and sausage are processed, they continue to add ingredients that only cause you inflammation. Try and eat organic, grass-fed meats and stay away from anything that has extra processing.

Bad Oils – Vegetable oils, frying oils, hydrogenated oils, and partially hydrogenated oils all wreak havoc on your body. They cause inflammation on your body and will leave you feeling worse. If you have to use an oil for cooking, it is best to stick to olive or coconut oil.

Processed Foods – Processed foods, packaged foods, and fast foods can lead to large amounts of inflammation. These have items that are not naturally occurring and are meant to make you want to come back for more. Always look at the ingredient list and if it has something in it that you cannot pronounce or do not know what it is, stay away.

Alcohol – Alcohol, as fun as you may find it, dehydrates and inflames your body. They put a burden on the liver and put a high sugar content in your body. If you must drink while trying to control your inflammation, make sure you do so in moderation and with consideration to sugar and calorie content.

It's important that you pay close attention to your body and how different foods affect you. This list is by no means comprehensive. Different people respond to different foods in different ways. The best way to follow the anti inflammatory diet is to pay close attention to how you are feeling. Just like the beginning of the book suggests, write it down. Right down how you feel and what you eat. You may find that there are foods that are not on this list that end up making you feel worse instead of better. It is important that you take good care of yourself as you embark on this journey. Keep a running list of foods you know you should avoid. On that same token, don't be afraid to spoil yourself *in moderation.* If you are constantly stressed out and battling your cravings to an extent that prevents you from being happy, you will not take to this diet well. Find foods that make you happy and make you feel good. If you have to splurge, make it occasional and make it small. Stress only increases inflammation and prevents your body from focusing on what you need it to focus on.

Chapter 5
Food You Should Be Eating

Just as there are foods that have inflammatory effects, there are foods that have anti-inflammatory properties. Add plenty of these foods to your diet to make yourself feel better. Working to eat these items will make you feel better, reduce inflammation, help reverse aging, reduce pain, and give you more energy.

Water – Staying hydrated is one of the most important aspects of your health. There is more about this in chapter three. You don't have to just drink water. You can drink plain hot tea, or iced tea, black coffee, and other water based drinks; just make sure that these drinks do not have added sugar or processed ingredients.

Oily or Fatty Fish – Oily fish is well known as a strong healthy tool. Make sure you keep this one in your arsenal. Salmon, tuna, mackerel, and sardines are high in omega-3 fatty acids. These fatty acids fight unnecessary inflammation in the body. They can help you stay healthy. If you have a hard time eating fish, try taking a fish-oil supplement.

Whole Grains – Whole grains are worlds better for you than the refined grains that are warned about in the last chapter. Rather than eating white breads, cereals, rice, and pasta, eat whole grains. This proper form of fiber is known for reducing levels of harmful toxins in your body that cause inflammation and keep you from feeling your best. Make sure you look for foods with whole grain as the first ingredient and without refined or processed sugar.

Dark Leafy Greens – Dark leafy greens are a fantastic source of vitamin E. This vitamin is well known for aiding in inflammation. Dark leafy greens protect your body against toxins and harmful things that will make you feel worse. Get your anti-inflammatory properties from your favorite dark, leafy greens such as kale, spinach, collard greens, and broccoli.

Nuts – Nuts are a great source of healthy fats and are proven to help reduce inflammation. They, along with fatty fish, are well known in the Mediterranean diet. This diet is proven to help reduce inflammation. Make sure you enjoy your nuts in moderation, you do not want to have too much of a good thing. The best nuts you can snack on and include in your meals are almonds, which are high in fiber. However, all nuts are high in antioxidants which help keep you healthy and well taken care of.

Tomatoes – Tomatoes are extremely versatile and make a meal wonderful. Tomatoes are also very good for you and can help fight inflammation. They are high in antioxidants and low in bad sugars.

Peppers – Have you ever had a pain cream that has capsaicin in it? This fun ingredient comes from peppers and is known to help fight pain and inflation. However, this inflation fighting food may not be for everyone. Keep an eye on how you feel when you eat peppers. Make sure you take it easy if you are feeling worse.

Beets and Beetroot Juice – The bright red color of this vegetable indicates that it has a lot of vitamin C and antioxidants. It is known to help with inflammation as well as pain and uncomfortable digestion. Keep an eye out for brightly colored vegetables like beets; their bright color indicates their good nutrition sources. Keep away from starchy veggies like potatoes and corn.

Berries and Raisins – This fantastic snacking item is high in antioxidants and can give you what you need to keep inflammation at bay. They also fight free radicals which will help keep you healthy.

Beans – Beans are packed with anti-inflammatory botanicals and can be used in several different recipes and are also known to help keep you full. Use these protein packed items to help you on your journey to feeling better and losing weight.

Ginger – Ginger does more than keep nausea at bay. It can help fight inflammation and stomach issues as well. Are you reading this book because you need help with digestion? Make sure you introduce a good amount of ginger in your diet.

Sweet Potatoes – In moderation, this food will not only help keep inflammation down, but it will help keep your blood sugar at bay.

Tea – Tea can help you do more than just add hydration. Sure, if you drink tea, you will help your own hydration out, but you can do more for yourself. You can introduce calming herbs into your body that can help reduce inflammation. Not only does tea help to keep inflammation at bay, but it can help keep you relaxed and calm which is another key element to keeping your inflammation at bay.

The anti-inflammatory diet is a lot about taking care of yourself and paying attention. Pay attention to how you feel compared with what you are eating. Start by following the guide of this book, but tailor the diet to yourself and how you feel. Unfortunately, I cannot give you the exact guide because every person is different and every person reacts to inflammatory foods differently. If you get in the habit of writing everything down, you will start to know what is affecting you. Don't worry if it does not work out at first, eventually you will get into a groove and you will figure it out. Following the anti inflammatory diet is committing to making a good life change that will leave you feeling so much better: you will lose weight, have more energy, reverse your own signs of aging, and most importantly, reduce inflammation.

Chapter 6

Time to Relax!

A really important aspect of reducing your inflammation is reducing your stress. If you are stressed out and worried about stuff, your body will not be able to help you heal. Adding stress and unrest to your life adds more distress. Studies show that people who are calm, relaxed, and less stressed tend to have better digestion and health. There are several methods of calming down and reducing stress that we will discuss here. Adjusting your diet alone might help you feel less stressed. If you are less worried about how you are feeling, you are going to end up adding more positivity to your life. Try some of these techniques to keep yourself less stressed and calmed down.

Meditation – If you are having trouble with stress, mediation may be a good way to take care of yourself. Many people find meditation a good practice to keep them calm. You can try it the simple way, or even research and try more advanced tactics. Start slow. Find a comfortable position. Make the room quiet or give yourself some calming meditation music to listen to. Clear your brain and calm down. Focus on your breathing. Meditation is not for everyone, but it may just make you feel better and give you the calmness you need to avoid some of your stresses and issues.

Breathing – If you don't have the time to mediate. At least give yourself a chance to focus on your breathing. Take a few deep breaths. Give yourself a calming break. Breath in for five counts and out for five counts. Make sure you are breathing deep from your belly and not in a shallow manner from your chest. Even something as simple as focusing on your breathing can give you a huge edge up on your anti-inflammatory journey.

Yoga – Yoga is a time honored tradition that has often helped many people. The awesome part about yoga is that it is both relaxing and exercise at the same point. It can help you stay relaxed and limber. There are several simple guides to doing yoga available online. You can even take classes. Many studies show that yoga can help you take care of yourself both on the inside and the outside.

Coloring – *What? Coloring can help me with my diet?* Sure it can! The new trend of coloring can make a huge difference in your life. It gives you the opportunity to calm down and focus on a singular task. Make sure you take the time to use coloring as a relaxing exercise.

Journaling – As was written at the beginning of the book, journaling can really help you a lot. Take the time to write down how you feel. You do not have to just stick to writing about how you feel about the diet and journey you are taking. You can take the time to write about your entire day. Use this both as a de-stressing tool and a strong indication of how you are feeling. Write down what you eat and how you feel about what you ate, and write about how your day went. This is a good way to identify the every day stresses that are preventing you from taking care of yourself.

Stress is such a mean monster. It can wreak havoc on your internal system and how you take care of yourself. When you are stressed, it is easier to break and eat foods that you know you should not. When you eat these foods that cause inflammation in your body, your body sends you signals that makes you want to eat more of these foods that inflame your body. Take care of your body and your body will take care of you.

Chapter 7
Thirty One Delicious Recipes

Lemon Pepper Salmon with Quinoa

Salmon is known to help fight inflammation with its awesome Omega-3 and good fat content. If you enjoy salmon, eat plenty of it, but make sure you prepare it right. Don't cook your salmon in vegetable oil or fats; that isn't good for you. Instead, you should use coconut oil or olive oil. These oils also add an extra inflammation-fighting aspect to your healthy meal. Quinoa is a whole grain and has plenty of different varieties available. This ancient grain is known to be healthy and helps keep you full and happy longer; not only does it have a great fiber content, but it has a great protein content as well. You can buy some already seasoned or you can add your seasoning. Of course, the best course of action is to season your quinoa, that way you make sure you do not have a bunch of extra processed ingredients. Pair this meal with a leafy green that will also help take care of you like spinach or broccoli.

Ingredients:

2 Salmon filets with skin

1 Tbsp. Olive Oil

4 Tbsp. Lemon Pepper Seasoning

2 Tbsp. Garlic Powder or 1 Tbsp. fresh garlic

½ cup of quinoa – unprepared

Begin by preparing your quinoa. There are many different varieties of quinoa, and some have different preparation processes. It is best to follow the directions that come with it. Most quinoas need a few minutes to sit and soak in the water. When you get to this stage, add your seasoning. You can put a bit of salt, or any form of seasoning you think will taste good.

Now it is time to move on to your salmon. Heat a skillet over medium heat then add olive oil. Put a generous amount of lemon pepper and garlic on the flesh side of the salmon. Place the salmon in the skillet skin side up. Once you see that the salmon has cooked ½ way through, remove it from the heat and flip it over. Allow the salmon to sit, covered, for about ten minutes. This allows the cooking process to finish.

Add your favorite veggies and you have a great anti-inflammatory meal!

Slow Cooker Stuffed Peppers

Slow cooker meals are an awesome way to come home to dinner already prepared. Do you have a busy week ahead of you? Throw a few slow cooker meals together ahead of time and put them in the freezer. Take it out to thaw the night before you want to eat it, throw it in the slow cooker in the morning, and you have yourself dinner that evening. Slow cookers are a great way to keep any harmful oven-toxins out of your food. They cook in a much cleaner, slower way.

Ingredients:

4 Bell Peppers

1 Tbsp. Olive Oil

1 small can of green chile

Unrefined salt (to taste)

½ lb. of ground turkey

1 can organic unsalted black beans

1 tomato

2 Cloves of Garlic, minced

Start by sautéing everything but your bell peppers in a pan over medium heat. Turkey first, then the rest of the ingredients. You are doing this to make sure that your turkey meat is cooked. If you place the raw turkey in the slow cooker, there is a change it will not finish cooking when the rest of the ingredients do. You don't want to risk getting your family sick. Instead, this will make you a nice mixture to put inside of your bell peppers.

If you are freezing this meal, you have two options here. You can either freeze the filling that you have just sautéed and add it to the bell peppers later, or you can add it to the bell peppers now and freeze them all together. Just make sure that if you are freezing this meal to slow cook at a later date that you allow the filling to cool completely to room temperature before you put it in the freezer.

Cut the tops off of your bell peppers and take out the insides. If you want to add a little extra kick to your meal, you can add a few seeds to your sauté, but the green chile should do a good job of adding spice and flavor already. Fill your peppers with the filling, and place in your slow cooker. Add enough water to cover ½ of the peppers and make sure your peppers stay upright. Cook on low for eight hours or high for four hours and you have yourself a fantastic meal.

Cashew Chicken Stir Fry

It's really easy to want to splurge on Chinese take-out, but once you learn how easy it is to make a quick stir-fry yourself, you may think twice before picking up your phone. By doing this yourself, you can create an awesome meal that you, your friends, and family will love, but that is not the only benefit. Take out generally has gobs of sodium, sugar, and MSG. These deadly devils will keep you far away from any of your anti-inflammatory goals. They will make you sick and keep your body from taking care of itself. However, if you use the right ingredient, you can actually turn this meal into one that will help you stick to your goals and take care of yourself.

Ingredients:

½ cup raw cashews, coarsely chopped

1 pound organic skinless chicken breast, cut into small bite sized pieces

2 Tbsp. unrefined, organic sesame oil

2 Tbsp. rice wine or rice wine vinegar

1 Tbsp. raw honey

4 cloves garlic, crushed

1 Tbsp. ginger, grated

1 onion, chopped

4 large carrots, peeled and cut

2 red bell peppers, seeded sliced thin

1 small can (5 ounces) water chestnuts, drained and chopped

2-3 Tbsp. organic, gluten-free soy sauce

½ cup green onions, sliced

3 cups black rice, brown rice, or quinoa cooked

Heat a large skillet over medium heat and cook your chicken. Once your chicken is finished, add your onions and allow them to cook for a minute. Place the rest of your vegetables into the pan and sauté everything together. Add the cashews, sesame oil, rice wine, honey, garlic, and ginger to your pan. Allow to simmer at a low heat for several minutes, stirring often. Make sure that everything gets sautéed and cooked into the sauce. Serve this over black rice, brown rice, or quinoa. It is easy to substitute some of the ingredients on this list for their less than healthy counterparts, but keep in mind that this will affect you feel.

Beans and Rice

Beans can be categorized into various forms such as lentils, kidney beans, black beans, navy beans, soy beans, and peanuts, and they all fall into a category of edible seeds that grow in pods called legumes. Most beans are low in sodium, calories, and they contain low-fat content. They are an excellent source of dietary fiber and some important complex carbohydrate, and they are moderately rich in fatty acids that are essential for your intake. At times, healing and strengthening your digestive tracts may be needed for you to get the best out of this food without experiencing any discomfort in your intestines. They are very vital in an anti-inflammatory diet due to their low ranking status on the glycemic scale; that is they prevent the inflammatory and hunger-inducing rise in your body's blood sugar level peculiar to highly processed foods and sugary foods. Beans can be used as ingredients in sauces and dips and can also be taken alongside dishes like high-protein salads, winter stews, etc.

Ingredients:

One teaspoon of olive oil

Two cloves of minced garlic

A chopped onion

½ cup of raw brown rice to be cooked in a rice cooker

A can of black beans

A cup of chicken broth and a vegetable broth

Turkey bacon (optional)

Add a teaspoon of olive oil in a stockpot and heat it up over medium heat. Add the two cloves of minced garlic, turkey bacon, and the chopped onion and cook over medium heat for about four minutes. Add the cooked brown rice and sauté for an additional two minutes. At this point, add a cup of vegetable broth and boil all together. Cover the stockpot and reduce the heat for about ten minutes, then add a can of black beans with an extra option of adding vegetables, and heat thoroughly. This delicious dish can be taken as dinner, and the leftover can be kept in a small container to be taken to work the following day.

Black-Eyed Peas and Spinach

Ingredients

Two teaspoons of olive oil

Two cloves of peeled garlic

A can of black-eyed peas

A moderately sized chopped onion

A bag of organic spinach

Lemon juice

Salt and Pepper

Two teaspoons of unroasted, raw, chopped almonds or a handful of dried cranberries.

Add two teaspoons of olive oil in a wide skillet or a steep-sided frying pan and apply medium heat for up to four minutes. Add a moderately-sized chopped onion and two cloves of peeled garlic and sauté over medium heat for an additional two minutes. Add a can of black eyed peas and cook, making sure you stir regularly for about five minutes until the beans are well heated. Lower the heat level, stir in a bag of organic spinach, cover and cook until the organic spinach has wilted down to the right standard of the black-eyed peas. As soon as it has wilted, stir again inside the skillet to ensure the organic spinach and the black eyed peas are evenly mixed, then remove from heat. Thoroughly Heat the olive oil, onion, and garlic in a large pan or wok for two to four minutes over medium heat, then add the black-eyed peas and stir to coat. Cook while occasionally stirring for about five minutes until the beans are heated through. Lower the heat, add the spinach and cover until the spinach has wilted (a large bag of spinach will wilt down to be the right proportion for the black eyed peas). Stir one more time in the wok to evenly mix the spinach and peas. Cook for about two minutes, then remove from heat. Season with salt, pepper, and lemon juice after serving.

Sesame Soba Noodles

Ingredients:

Eight oz. of soba noodles

A clove of minced garlic

A tablespoon of fresh lime juice

¼ teaspoon of ginger root

Three green chopped onions

¼ teaspoon of ground cumin

Two tablespoons of sesame seed butter

Three tablespoons of warm water

1/8 teaspoon of salt

Six tablespoons of vegetable or chicken broth

Three tablespoons of sesame water

Sauté the soba noodles by following its guidelines and package directions until cooked. Place the cooked soba noodles inside a relatively cold water for a few seconds to help prevent the noodles from sticking together, then get rid of the cold water and return the noodles to a serving plate. Lift the noodles and turn it over using two tablespoons of broth and keep them in the refrigerator to chill. During this process, add a clove of minced garlic, a tablespoon of fresh lime juice, sesame seed butter, gingerroot, ¼ teaspoon of cumin, sesame seed butter, salt, and water. Leave the pasta for a while till it reaches room temperature, then toss with the sesame sauce until well coated. Stir in the remaining chicken or vegetable broth and garnish with three green onions and sesame seeds. Additionally, include a sautéed chicken or some hard-boiled eggs that have been sliced to increase the protein content of this dish and eat.

Banana Nut Pancakes

Ingredients:

A teaspoon of cinnamon

1½ cups of rice flour

A cup of hazelnut milk

2½ tablespoons of non-aluminum baking powder

1/3 cup of chopped pecans

¼ cup of brown rice syrup

¾ cup of water, and two tablespoons of water in two different places

Canola oil to be added in a griddle

A cup of mashed banana

Heat up your griddle to around 350°F. Add 1½ cups of rice flour, one teaspoon of cinnamon, baking powder, chopped pecans in a big bowl and mix thoroughly. Also, add a cup of hazelnut milk, ¼ cup of brown rice syrup, and water, stir thoroughly until well mixed. Mix all the wet ingredients with the dry ingredients and stir thoroughly. Stir in a cup of the mashed banana until it has mixed thoroughly with the ingredients. Add a tablespoon of canola oil in the preheated griddle. Carefully pour the mixed ingredients in the griddle and carve out four pancakes. Sauté until bubbles appear in the middle of the pancake. Flip the four pancakes over and cook for an additional two minutes. Serve immediately.

Black Bean Avocado Dip

Ingredients:

½ cup of well drained and properly rinsed canned black beans

A clove of minced garlic

Two tablespoons of minced red onion

½ cup of already cooked brown rice

A large ripe avocado

Salt and pepper for seasoning

Place ½ cup of rinsed black beans in a bowl and heat in a Microwave for about a minute until the beans soft, and cool. Pitt the avocado very smoothly and roughly mix two tablespoons of minced red onion and a clove of minced garlic. Stir in the cooked rice into the avocado mixture, add the cooked black beans and mix gently to avoid breaking up the black beans too much. Season with salt and pepper, then serve at room temperature or when chilled.

Amaranth Porridge

This gluten-free "grain" is easily digestible and contains Manganese which is very essential in preventing and repairing damages in ligaments and joints.

Ingredients:

Two cups if filtered water

A tablespoon of raw honey

A teaspoon of cinnamon

¼ cup of pumpkin seeds or hemp

2/3 cup of whole-grain amaranth

½ cup of dried cranberries or blueberries

A medium sized chopped pear

Add whole-grain amaranth together with water in a skillet and cover very tightly with a lid. Heat up until it reaches boiling point, then lower the heat level and simmer for about thirty minutes. Ensure you stir at ten minutes interval to prevent the whole-grain amaranth from sticking to the pot while they absorb the water in the skillet. Remove the skillet from heat and stir in other ingredients like a tablespoon of raw honey, cinnamon, and the pumpkin seeds. Add a medium sized pear or blueberries as toppings and serve when hot. The leftovers should be placed in a container with a tight-fitting cover and kept for the next day.

Mango Rice Pilaf

Ingredients:

A teaspoon of canola oil

¼ cup of thinly sliced green onion

¼ teaspoon of salt

1/8 teaspoon of pepper

Two cups of finely chopped fresh baby spinach

1/8 teaspoon of dried thyme

¼ cup of neatly sliced fresh mushrooms

1/3 cup of sautéed wild rice

¾ cup of diced fresh or chilled mango

1/8 cup of roughly chopped sliced almonds

1 1/3 cups of sautéed brown rice (basmati)

1/8 cup of broth

Add a teaspoon of canola oil in a big stockpot and heat moderately. Add the neatly sliced mushrooms and sauté for about five minutes until the color becomes golden brown and crisp. Add two cups of fresh baby spinach and cook for two minutes until it becomes wilted. Add the wild rice, brown rice, dried thyme, pepper, green onions, broth, sliced almonds, and salt, then mix thoroughly. Add mango and heat all together. Serve immediately.

Guacamole

Ingredients:

Two pitted and peeled avocados

About 1/8 to 1/4 cup extra virgin olive oil

Fresh cilantro

½ cup of lime juice

Sea salt

Beat the peeled avocado and extra virgin olive oil with a fork and whip carefully inside a mixing bowl till it gets roughly smooth. Fold this roughly smooth mixture in the cilantro, sea salt, and lime juice. Additional ingredients like ground cumin and finely chopped green onions can be added to increase yield and modify taste.

White Bean Spread or Dip

Ingredients:

Eight oz. of sautéed canned white beans

A small bunch of leafy green arugula

Two tablespoons of oil

Two tablespoons of vegetable stock or chicken

Two tablespoons of minced garlic

A tablespoon of capers

Salt

Pepper

Open the white beans with a can opener, drain
and thoroughly rinse through while they
beans are still in the can. Peel off the garlic
and press very hard to squeeze. Carefully
remove the stems of the leafy green arugula
and rinse thoroughly. Add the remaining

ingredients (excluding salt) in a blender and blend at high speed. Season the blended mixture with pepper and salt and mix carefully in the arugula. This dish can either be used to garnish chicken or taken as a vegetable dip.

Hearty Sweet Potatoes

A large sweet potato that has been cut into different cubes

Two tablespoons of olive oil

Two tablespoons of butter

¼ teaspoon of cumin

A can of cannellini beans

Finely chopped fresh parsley

Chopped onion

Sea salt

In a medium-sized saucepan, cook the sweet potato in butter over medium heat until it becomes soft. Add chopped onion and cook for an additional three minutes until the onion softens. Open the canned cannellini beans with a can opener, add and heat through. Add ¼ teaspoon of cumin, then season with salt and pepper. Remove the saucepan from the heat and add the finely chopped fresh parsley, lightly spray with olive oil, then serve.

Hummus

Ingredients:

¼ cup of chicken or vegetable broth

Five tablespoons of lemon juice

Three cloves of minced garlic

Three tablespoons of Tahini

Two tablespoons of olive oil

Sixteen oz. of canned garbanzo beans

Add all the listed ingredients in a large mixing cup of your blender and blend at high speed. Pulse repeatedly till the mixture becomes smooth. This meal is mostly served in a small bowl after it has been lightly sprayed with two tablespoons of olive oil sprinkled with paprika. Garnish with fresh parsley and eat.

Chicken in Garlic, Shallots and Herbs

Ingredients:

Four oz. of chicken per person

A boneless or skinless chicken breast or ¼ cup of two chicken thighs

Two tablespoons of olive oil

Peeled cloves of garlic

Six peeled shallots

Salt

Pepper

Herbs of your preference(you can choose any between fresh parsley, thyme, sage, etc.)

Heat up your oven to about 375°F. While this is ongoing, add salt and pepper seasoning to the chicken and toss with two tablespoons of olive oil.   Deep-fry the chicken in a medium sized skillet on both sides until the color becomes brown. After this has been done, remove the browned chicken from the skillet and add shallots, garlic, herbs, and the remaining olive oil. Cover the skillet firmly and bake for at least an hour, then you are done.

Superfood Smoothie

Ingredients:

An avocado and a banana

A handful of baby spinach leaves or rocket leaves

A tablespoon of bee pollen

A tablespoon of agave nectar/raw honey

A tablespoon of maca powder

Two cups of pure water

A cup of ice

A tablespoon of raw cacao powder

A tablespoon of barley grass powder

Add all the listed ingredients in a blender and blend at high speed, until the mixture becomes smooth and runny. Serve and drink instantly.

Limas and Spinach

Ingredients:

Two cups of frozen lima beans

½ cup of chopped onions

A tablespoon of vegetable oil

A tablespoon of distilled vinegar

1/8 teaspoon of black pepper

Four cups of thoroughly rinsed leaf spinach

A cup of fennel

A tablespoon of raw chives

¼ cup of low-sodium chicken broth

Bring lima beans to boil in unsalted water for about ten minutes, then drain. Pour a tablespoon of vegetable oil in a skillet, add chopped onions and fennel, then cook over medium heat. Add chicken broth and lima beans, cover with a tight-fitting lid and sauté for about two minutes. Add leaf spinach, cover and cook for about two minutes until the leaf spinach wilts, then add distilled vinegar and pepper. Replace the lid and cook over low heat for up to thirty seconds. Sprinkle the dish with fresh chives and serve.

Tuna Salad

Ingredients:

½ cup of chopped raw celery

6½ tablespoons of low-fat mayonnaise

1/3 cup of chopped green onions

Two cans of water pack tuna

Thoroughly rinse and drain tuna for about five minutes. Split with a fork. Add chopped green onions, chopped raw celery, low-fat mayonnaise and mix thoroughly. This anti-inflammatory dish can be great for a sandwich or lunchtime salad plate.

Almond Blueberry Orzo

Ingredients:

½ cup of blueberries

½ teaspoon of cinnamon

1½ tablespoon of almond butter

1½ teaspoons of vanilla extract

½ cup of pasta orzo

½ cup of low-fat milk

2/3 cup of non-fat Greek yogurt

Stevia sweetener

Follow the label guidelines and directions to prepare the pasta. When done, drain the pasta and place in a saucepan or skillet. Add low-fat milk and stir very well. Cook over a relatively low heat for a while. Add half of the blueberries, cinnamon, almond butter, and vanilla and bring to boil. Remove the saucepan or skillet from heat and stir in the remaining blueberries. Split into two different bowls and top with non-fat Greek yogurt, and serve.

Blueberry Cottage Cheese

Ingredients:

Five teaspoons of silvered almonds

½ cups of fresh or frozen blueberries

½ cup of non-sugary applesauce

A teaspoon of extra virgin olive oil

¾ cup of reduced fat cottage cheese

Add the non-sugary applesauce, cottage cheese, and extra virgin olive oil in a bowl and mix thoroughly. Stir in blueberries and almonds.

Apple Jumble Zinger

Ingredients:

A teaspoon of olive oil

A cup of strawberries

Two tablespoons of raw almonds

Six hard-boiled egg whites without the yolk
from the previous night.

1½ tablespoons of raw ginger

A medium-sized apple

Hard-boil six eggs and get rid of the yolks a
night before preparing this meal. Add all the

ingredients together in a blender cup and blend at high speed, until the mixture becomes chunky.

Jicama, Orange and Avocado Salad

Ingredients:

Four cups of peeled Jicama

Two tablespoons of minced fresh cilantro

Two peeled oranges

1/3 cup of fresh squeezed orange juice

½ avocado cut into cubes

¼ teaspoon of salt

Two tablespoons of lime juice

A cup of chopped Perdue or leftover boneless and skinless chicken breast

Toss jicama with two tablespoons of lime juice, salt, and fresh squeezed orange juice. Allow the mixture to marinate for about three hours, then add the two peeled oranges, cubed avocado, and fresh cilantro to jicama. Toss the jicama and stir to coat. This ideal lunch can be topped with chicken breast before serving.

Mediterranean Salad with Fusilli

Ingredients:

¼ cup of chopped cucumber

Two tablespoons of fresh squeezed lemon juice

Black pepper

Oregano

½ teaspoon of olive oil

One ounce of low-fat feta

Eight cherry tomatoes cut into halves

½ cup of pasta fusilli

Three chopped olives

Prepare the pasta by following the directions and guidelines on the package and let it cool. While cooling the pasta, cut the cucumber and tomato into equal chunks and add to the prepared pasta together with other listed ingredients. This is very easy to prepare and goes well with lunch or dinner.

Mexi Chicken Chili

Ingredients:

Two ounces of cooked skinless chicken breast

Two chopped tomatoes

½ chopped onion

Four chopped black olives

One teaspoon of olive oil

One tablespoon of low-fat shredded mozzarella

¼ cup of black beans

2/3 cup of salsa

One teaspoon of chili powder

Add all the listed ingredients in a microwave-safe bowl and mix thoroughly. Place the bowl containing the mixture in a microwave and heat until it is warm. You may want to include some fresh parsley or cilantro for a bit of added freshness and drizzle with a teaspoon of olive oil.

Midday Omelet

Ingredients:

A tablespoon of sliced almonds

1/3 teaspoon of olive oil

Two tablespoons of shredded mozzarella cheese

Six sliced olives

A cup of non-sugary applesauce

Two slices of chopped Canadian bacon

¼ cup of Salsa

½ cup of egg whites

Add olive oil in a sprayed skillet and heat it
up. Add ½ cup of egg whites and cook until it
is slightly done. Add shredded mozzarella
cheese, Canadian bacon, and sliced olives.
Toss and constantly turn until sautéed. This
omelet can be served with Salsa with sliced
almonds and applesauce as dessert.

Raspberry Balsamic Reduction for Salmon

Ingredients:

½ cup of balsamic vinegar

½ cup of raspberries

¼ teaspoon of pepper

½ teaspoon of coconut crystals

½ teaspoon of salt

One tablespoon of chopped basil

Three tablespoons of olive oil

A tablespoon of chopped fresh parsley

Add three tablespoons of olive oil together with balsamic vinegar, raspberries, coconuts crystals, salt, and pepper in a medium-sized saucepan and cook over medium heat. As soon as the mixture shrinks, add fresh parsley and basil. Remove the saucepan from the heat source and allow to cool. Drizzle a little quantity over baked, grilled, or fried fish to make a delicious meal and eat.

Mango Avocado Salsa

Ingredients:

Two diced avocados

One ripe diced mango

Lemon or lime juice, according to your choice

A finely chopped small shallot

Two cloves of minced garlic

Neatly chopped fresh cilantro

Salt and pepper

Add all ingredients together in a mixing bowl and mix thoroughly. Keep the leftover salsa in a refrigerator and take the next day.

Almond Banana Shake

Ingredients:

Two bananas

Two cups of almond milk

½ teaspoon of vanilla extract

¼ teaspoon of nutmeg

Add all the listed ingredients in a blender and blend at high speed until it becomes smooth. Sprinkle ¼ teaspoon of nutmeg on its top and serve immediately.

Caribbean Cooler

Ingredients:

¾ teaspoon of vanilla extract

½ cup of non-sugary pineapple juice

¾ teaspoon of almond extract

1½ teaspoons of coconut crystals

½ cup of almond milk

Add all ingredients together in a blender and blend thoroughly to become smooth. Pour into different glasses and serve.

Pesto Mushrooms

Ingredients:

Twenty button mushrooms or four portobello mushrooms

½ cup of pine nuts

One cup of walnuts

A teaspoon of salt

Three cups of basil

½ cup of olive oil

Lemon juice substitutes (about two tablespoons)

Three cloves of minced garlic

Thoroughly rinse the mushrooms and stem them neatly. Put the washed mushrooms on a serving plate. Add the remaining ingredients together and blend at high speed until the mixture becomes smooth. Fill up the mushrooms in a serving plate with pesto and serve immediately.

Black Olive Tapenade

Ingredients:

Lemon juice (about two tablespoons)

½ cup of olive oil

Three cloves of garlic

Fresh parsley(about one small handful)

Sea salt (about a teaspoon)

Pitted black olives of about three cups

Except for the black olives, blend the listed ingredients above at high speed until it becomes smooth. Add olives to the smooth mixture and beat until well chopped. Serve using a dip with flax crackers.